MW01631742

ADVANCED PRAISE

Reading this booklet is extremely informative and serves as a vital tool/resource that is truly needed in any community during one of the toughest times in a person's life—death. Although death is inevitable, dealing with it and how loved ones navigate the hardship looks different for everyone. This booklet certainly eases some of the burdens of managing practical matters and provides a step-by-step guide to make an extremely tough and emotional time much easier to navigate. This is truly a must-buy!

– Najah Joseph

I love that this booklet is concise and easy to understand and the resources are accessible.

– Gail Kennard.

End *of* Life

HAVING THE DIFFICULT CONVERSATIONS

TARYN L. SIDDIQ

END OF LIFE
Having the Difficult Conversations

For information about special discounts for bulk purchases, please write eolconvos@tarynlsiddiq.com.

www.TarynlSiddiq.com

Produced by Book Power Publishing
Book Power books may be purchased for educational, business, or sales promotional use.

FIRST EDITION
PRINTED IN THE UNITED STATES OF AMERICA

Ebook ISBN: 978-1-964965-06-2
Paperback ISBN: 978-1-964965-05-5

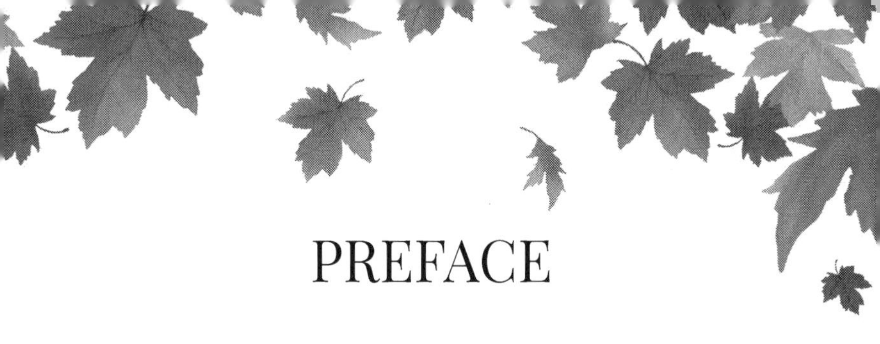

PREFACE

I've had difficult conversations my entire life, but as a Clinical Social Worker, they've become even more challenging. I often meet families and patients who haven't given much thought to what they would want at the end of their lives, let alone discussed it with their loved ones, doctors, friends, or even acquaintances. Many only begin to consider these decisions as they age, face an illness, or confront their own mortality when others pass. Most people, however, avoid the topic entirely, hoping they won't have to address it.

Questions like, *"Do they have an Advance Directive or Living Will?" "Do they want to remain on a ventilator or life support?" "Do they want nutrition or hydration?"* often go unasked.

Families are asked—or left wondering: *"What kind of life did your loved one have?" "Do you know what they would want?" "Have they ever mentioned their wishes?" "Do they want a funeral, memorial, or cremation?" "How do they want to be remembered?" "Do they want a celebration of life or simply an obituary notice?"*

As the saying goes in a famous movie, *"Get busy living or get busy dying."* This sentiment echoes the wisdom of Prophet Muhammad (Peace and Blessings Be Upon Him), who said, *"Live as if it's your last day, and live as if you'll live forever."* We should always prepare for death because no one knows when their time will come.

Personally, I've become more aware of death after experiencing significant loss—family, friends, and a few colleagues. At times, these losses have shaken me to my core. Unexpected death can leave you so disoriented that it's hard to process. When illness is involved, you may have some time to prepare yourself, but who is preparing the person who is actively dying?

This booklet is a brief guide to help you think about these matters as life goes on, regardless of your faith. It's easy to brush it off, telling yourself, *"I'll think about this tomorrow,"* or *"I'll complete my Advance Directive or Will tomorrow,"* or *"I'll have that conversation tomorrow."* But for many, tomorrow never comes, and their next of kin is left to figure it all out.

ACKNOWLEDGMENTS

I must begin by acknowledging Almighty God, whose guidance has been my anchor throughout this journey. I am also deeply grateful to my patients, doctors, friends, colleagues, patient families, strangers, authors, films, life itself, and even myself for steering me toward spiritual healing in this profoundly human subject. Growth in this area demands facing one's own mortality with honesty, no matter how painful or frightening it may be. My experiences with loss have been my greatest teachers, and without them, I could not have written this book.

I never imagined that one of my life's journeys would involve writing about the end of life—a reality we all must face. The difficult conversations I've encountered so often in my personal and professional life have become a part of who I am, and I am grateful for the lessons they've brought. Who would have thought these moments would serve as my teachers, preparing me for my own difficult conversation with myself?

My deepest acknowledgment is to Almighty God, who placed this calling in my heart: to help others confront their mortality and find peace and closure, even as they prepare for the ultimate closure. As the saying goes (paraphrased), *"Don't be so focused on the loss of others that you forget to prepare for your own."*

Preparing

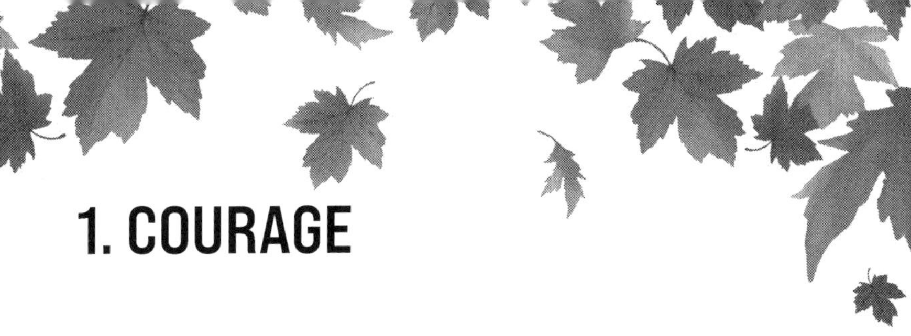

1. COURAGE

It takes nerve, strength, introspection, sensitivity, and true courage to face your own mortality. We're often so busy living that we don't pause to think about dying—there's always too much to do! Why dwell on it? Let's live in the moment and enjoy the life Almighty God has blessed us with. After all, if you're in your 20s, 30s, 40s, 50s, or even 60s, and you're healthy, why worry? You're living your best life!

But real courage also means having the insight, compassion, and empathy to acknowledge that life doesn't last forever and that preparation is a gift to those we leave behind. Why prepare? Because those who love you can't read your mind. In their grief and numbness, they'll already be navigating the pain of loss—should they also have to figure out what you would have wanted? Why should they be left to sift through papers, trying to locate your Advance Directive, Living Will, insurance documents, or passwords for bank accounts and emails? That's an unnecessary and overwhelming burden.

Courage means having those honest conversations with your loved ones—during family meetings, one-on-one talks, or gatherings—ensuring your wishes are clear. It's an act of love to relieve your family of the weight of uncertainty, allowing them to grieve without added stress.

Reflective Question:

Have I been courageous in my own preparations? Are there areas where I need more courage for myself and love ones?

____

____

____

____

What personal values or beliefs guide my understanding of COURAGE when facing the challenging decisions surrounding end-of- life care, and how do these values influence my choices for myself or my loved ones in these critical moments?

____

____

____

____

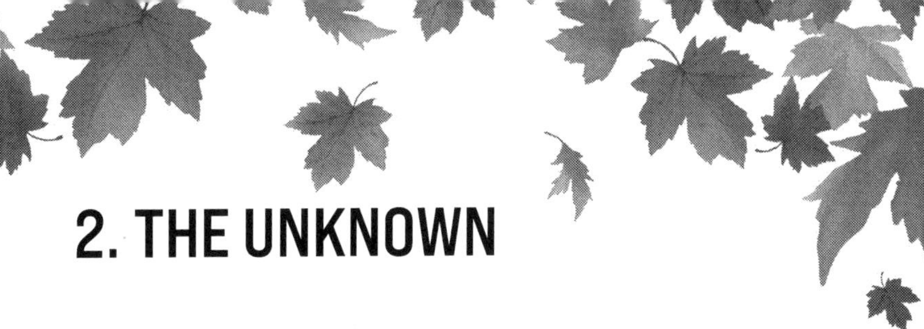

2. THE UNKNOWN

It's the unknown that often causes us to procrastinate and avoid facing reality. We don't know what we don't know. No one has come back to tell us what happens after death, so why confront it? For many, it feels easier to avoid the topic altogether.

Yet, those who approach life with a sense of spiritual awareness and consciousness understand that preparation is essential—no matter their faith or beliefs. The unknown can be unsettling, and we shy away from discussing it because it feels too heavy, too painful, or too final. We soothe ourselves with excuses: *"Not now." "It's not a good time." "I don't want to talk about it."* or *"Later."*

But avoidance doesn't change the fact that the unknown is inevitable. Preparing for it, however uncomfortable, is an act of care for ourselves and our loved ones. Facing the unknown head-on, with faith, curiosity, and strength, allows us to make thoughtful, informed decisions that ease the path for everyone involved.

Reflective Question:

How do my feelings about the UNKNOWN aspects of end-of-life decisions impact my ability to make informed choices for myself or my loved ones?

What steps can I take to transform the unknown into meaningful actions that bring clarity and peace to myself and my loved ones?

3. FEAR

Why is there fear? Some say that fear reflects a lack of faith. Without spiritual awareness, we can drift through life, uncertain of how our story will end. We all hope for a good ending—but what does that truly mean?

For many, a "good ending" represents a peaceful passing, free from suffering. But the truth is, we don't know what our final moments will be like. Our ideas about what constitutes a good ending vary, often shaped by our faith, beliefs, and personal experiences.

Reflective Question:

What specific fears arise for me when I think about end-of-life decisions? How do these fears shape the choices I make for myself or my loved ones?

____

____

____

____

4. ANGER

Who are we angry with? God, ourselves, family, or our loved one? The frustration often stems from not knowing how to handle that anger. As my 92year-old mother wisely says, 'Everyone has a day.' Once we recognize this, it's important to prepare ourselves and those we care about.

Reflective Question:

Am I angry? About what specifically?

____

____

____

____

How does this anger affect or influence my decision-making process relating to pain, impact on family or other areas?

____

____

____

____

Has this anger allowed me to be "stuck" or "frozen" in my ability to be helpful?

____

____

____

____

5. WHY?

Why not? Once you've had the difficult conversation and put the necessary documents and plans in place, navigating the end-of-life process becomes much easier for your family and loved ones. They will know exactly where to find important documents and who to call—whether it's an Imam, Rabbi, Priest, Minister, or Pastor, depending on your faith. They'll also have clarity on who handles your finances, obituary, burial arrangements, and any repast details, if desired.

By organizing these details in advance, you relieve your loved ones of unnecessary stress during a time of grief. Even in sorrow, they can focus on honoring your wishes rather than scrambling to figure out what you would have wanted. It's also wise to ensure that the secretary at your place of worship has up-to-date contact details for your next of kin, including phone numbers, emails, and addresses.

Reflective Question:

Have I taken steps to ensure my loved ones have clear guidance when the time comes? If not, what is holding me back?

____

____

____

____

What benefits do you receive having these end-of-life conversations?

____

____

____

____

6. COMING TO TERMS/PEACE

After it's all said and done, you can find peace in knowing you honored your loved one's wishes, allowing you, your family, and your departed loved one to rest peacefully. Yes, there will still be much to do in settling their affairs, but you'll be better prepared. Seeking bereavement counseling is always an option if you choose. Remember, there is no set timeline for grief—everyone grieves differently. Take all the time you need to honor your loved one's memory, knowing you fulfilled their desires.

As time moves on, certain experiences, memories, or even solitude may trigger feelings of sadness, tearfulness, withdrawal, and sometimes depression. This is normal. Telling someone to "get over it already," regardless of how long it's been, is insensitive and shows a lack of empathy. Often, it's better to simply be present, offer silent support, and pray for them, sharing words of encouragement when needed. Saying, "I know how you feel" can come across as disingenuous, especially if you don't. In any case, sincerity and honesty are always best.

Reflective Question:

How can you find peace in honoring your loved one's memory, and what steps can you take to ensure you are at peace with the process of grieving?

What comes to mind when you are COMING TO TERMS and seeking PEACE regarding your love ones end-of-life decision making process. What matters to you?

7. ACCEPTANCE/CONTENTMENT

Once the dust settles, time will bring a sense of acceptance and peace, knowing that having that difficult conversation was worth it, despite the pain. The discussions may have been uncomfortable, tense, or even emotional, yet thoughtful and sensitive. Ultimately, they prepared you for the inevitable moment when the loss could no longer be avoided.

Reflective Questions:

How did having that difficult conversation help you prepare for the inevitable loss? What steps can you take to find peace and contentment in this process, knowing that you were able to honor the conversation despite the discomfort?

____

____

____

____

How has this end-of-life process impacted you to the point of ACCEPTANCE/CONTENTMENT?

____

____

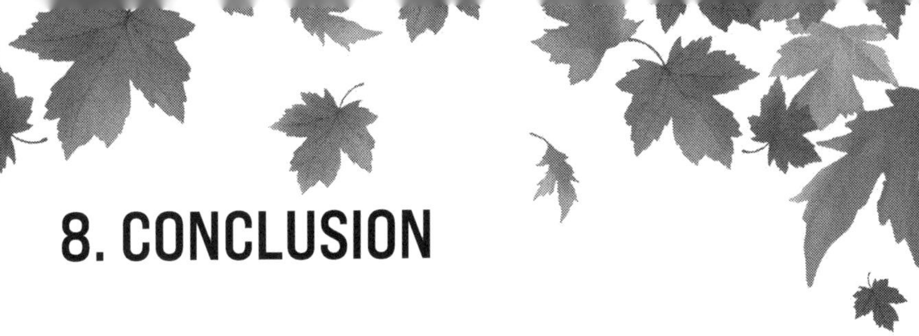

8. CONCLUSION

I pray that this booklet serves as a gentle reminder to take care of yourself and your loved ones. It encourages you to prepare and have those difficult conversations, so when the time comes, you can feel that it was all worth it and that you were fully prepared.

Reflective Question:

How can you begin preparing for those difficult conversations now, so you can approach them with peace and clarity when the time comes?

____

____

____

____

Have you been INTENTIONAL in this process? Why or why not?

____

____

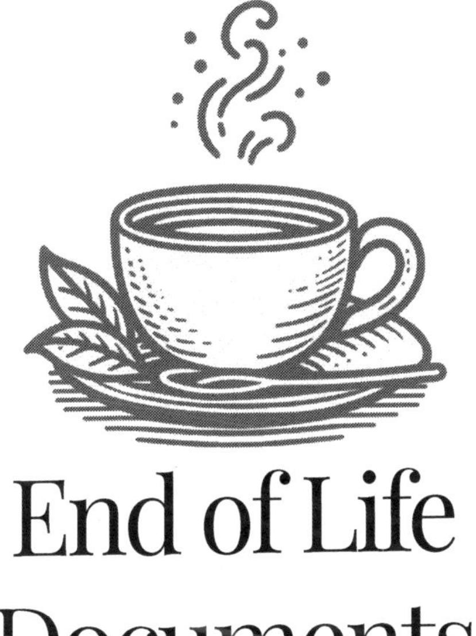

End of Life Documents

NEXT OF KIN (NOK) INFORMATION OR THE NOKBOX

(Found online at www.thenokbox.com). An organized approach to secure your life's details, such as accounts, possessions, social media presence, communities, passwords, etc.

WILL

A will is a legal document that, among other things, outlines where you want your assets to go after you die.

LIVING REVOCABLE TRUST

An arrangement set up through a legal document that gives someone the power to make decisions about another person's money or property held in the trust.

LIVING WILL

You outline your preferences about future healthcare treatments in case you are ever unable to communicate your wishes to doctors and loved ones.

DURABLE POWER OF ATTORNEY FOR HEALTHCARE (DPOA)

A legal document that allows someone to name a person to make medical decisions (not just at the end of life; this can apply to any medical condition) on their behalf if they are unable to do so. The person named to make decisions is called an agent or attorney-in-fact.

ADVANCE DIRECTIVES

A legal document that states a person's wishes about receiving medical care if that person is no longer able to make medical decisions due to a serious illness or injury. There are different types, e.g., Living Will, DPOA for Healthcare, and Do Not Resuscitate (DNR) Orders. The laws may be different for each state.

NOTIFICATION LIST

Prepare a notification list to ensure that everyone close to you is informed of your passing. This is especially helpful because your children, spouse, or close family may not know everyone significant in your life. You wouldn't want someone who is close to you to hear about your passing by chance. Here's how to create and maintain your notification list:

Who to include:

- Close friends
- Extended family members
- Professional colleagues
- Mentors or mentees
- Members of community or religious organizations

Details to provide:

- Full name
- Contact information (phone number, e-mail, or mailing address)
- Any notes on their relationship to you (Optional)

How to store the list:

- Save the document on a flash drive and/or upload your items to the "CLOUD".
- Keep it with other essential documents such as your will, trust, advance directives, burial wishes, and a list of key contacts (attorney, financial advisor).

Review and update regularly:

Review the list annually to add or remove names as necessary. This simple yet meaningful gesture can help ensure that everyone important to you is properly informed, reducing stress for your family and friends during a difficult time.

Thank You Gail Kennard for this thoughtful mention.

Addendum
The Islamic Perspective

THE ISLAMIC PERSPECTIVE

All Muslims should be buried within three days of death. When there appear to be exceptions or delays due to homicide or a pandemic, an Imam should be consulted and involved with the Coroner's Office to facilitate burial within this time frame.

The following questions should be discussed when **HAVING THE DIFFICULT CONVERSATIONS**:

1. Do you have life insurance?
2. Do you have a will?
3. Are you connected to a Muslim community? Who from that community would you like to wash and shroud your body?
4. Who has access to your personal paperwork, such as your life insurance policy and your will?
5. Does the Imam and two other members of your community have access to your family in the event of your death?
6. What provisions have you made financially to take care of your family after death? *GoFundMe and funeral fish fries are unacceptable.*
7. Muslims who have not planned for death and have not communicated with their non-Muslim family members about the Islamic End of Life Traditions will leave it up to them to make those decisions. Therefore, you might be cremated, not washed, or placed in a suit and tie instead of a shroud, or your funeral might be in a Christian church instead of a Masjid.

Start **HAVING THE DIFFICULT CONVERSATIONS** and **PLAN NOW!**

-The author extends appreciation to Na'im Hassan, who is also a contributor to this addendum.

About the author

Taryn is a Clinical Social Worker, Founder and President of the non-profit organization Muslimah Consultation Group, Inc. She is also a devoted wife, caregiver to her 92 years young mother, mother of 2 adult children, grandmother to 3 adult grandchildren, aunt to several, and now author.

Made in the USA
Columbia, SC
21 May 2025

58186106R00022